How Does He Do It? [Vol. 1]

Live Healthier, Stay Youthful, Be Happy!

Narc Narcisse

This book represents the ideas, research, and opinions of its author. It is not intended to be a substitute for the medical advice of a licensed physician. The readers should consult with their doctor for any matters related to their health, including starting a new diet or making changes to any current one. This book is presented as general advice on health care, and it contains information that is intended to help the readers be better informed consumers of health care. Always consult your doctor for your individual needs.

MENU

APPETIZER "Who The *Hell* is Narc Narcisse?" [PART I]......................1

Chapter 1: The Beginning… 3

MAIN COURSE "Why Do You Eat That Way?" 9

Chapter 2: My History with Food 11

Chapter 3: My Meals 15

Chapter 4: My Do's...22

Chapter 5: My Don'ts 30

DESSERT "Can I Have That Last Piece?"...35

Chapter 6: You Shouldn't Do That, You Should Do This 37

Chapter 7: My Final words 40

About The Author 43

PREFACE
This book is the result of two things.

First of all, for over a decade, people have been surprised when they find out how old I am. These people include strangers I meet at parties, at the gym, on vacation, and so on; but they also include people I know on a personal level, such as colleagues, athletes, students, parents, friends of friends, and sometimes even my younger friends—who simply assume I am their age. Now that I've crossed into my 40s, that surprise often turns into shock. I've had to show my ID on many occasions to prove my birth year—1977, baby! For some of my friends, it has become a source of entertainment to ask strangers to guess my age. What happens next is usually a barrage of questions about what my secrets are, how I am doing it, what I eat, what my workouts are, what products I use on my skin, what principles I adhere to, what my life philosophies are, and so forth.

Second of all, some of my friends have urged me to share my experiences via a blog, a book, a website, an Instagram page, a Facebook page, a YouTube channel, a podcast, or something of that nature; they claim I have something to offer...

"I do!"

With this book, I want to accomplish three things:

Inspire, Inform, Empower

ACKNOWLEDGEMENTS

I want to thank my parents. Without you, I wouldn't be the person I am today. You've always supported me, and you also gave me my genetics. Special shout out to my mom—*just because!* Bisous.

I want to thank the rest of my family: siblings, cousins, aunts, uncles, and so forth. I don't see you often, but know that I miss you all, and I'm always happy when we get together.

I want to thank my friends—i.e. my *chosen* family. I'm lucky to have you all in my life. I always look forward to conversing, hanging out, partying, traveling, and so on. Let the good times roll!

Special thanks to Dr. Mike L., my first roommate out of UCLA. More than a decade ago, you were the first person who suggested I write a book. At the time, I wasn't so sure about that. I didn't have a true vision yet, but you clearly saw something. Thanks!

Special thanks to my homies Rodrigue T., Taj B., and Jonah U.— my brothers from another mother. Friends for decades; you know me better than most. French-Caribbean, Indian-Scottish, and Nigerian-American; what a crew! In the past years, you guys also suggested I share my knowledge on various topics. Thanks for the advice and motivation!

Special thanks to Ananda D. and Sunny K. When I was writing this book, you both happened to be visiting Los Angeles—from Brazil and from Washington D.C. respectively—and when I mentioned the book, you both loved the idea. You had great enthusiasm, suggestions, and information that helped me tremendously. Obrigado!

Special thanks to Umar and Saouda N. It was great visiting you and your beautiful week-old baby girl, Sarah. When I mentioned the book, your faces lit up! When great friends are pumped like that, it makes it that much more motivating. You both had great insights and great ideas. Thanks!

Special thanks to Elizabeth P. and Peggy E. You were the first two people who knew about this book, and you gave me great positive energy to go for it. You also helped me with great ideas and were absolute superstars with your great editing skills. Thank you!

Special thanks to Başak E. Of the seven people that knew about this book, you were the last one to find out, but your energetic enthusiasm was amazing! After a rough week of writing, I knew I had to make some major changes. Your timely analysis, advice, ideas, and edits were spot on. You were truly the spark I needed. Two days after our conversation, the book was 95% done. Teşekkürler!

And last but not least, a HUGE thanks to my former high school Physics student Preston M. (Brentwood School 2005/06). It was fun running into you, David P., Patrick O., and others at the Bungalow in Santa Monica—Labor Day weekend, 2017. It's always good to catch up with my former students and athletes. As we reminisced about the good old days, you repeated how young I looked and how I hadn't changed since 2005. You suggested I create a website to reveal my "secrets" of youth—that was the clincher! I thought about that for the rest of the day, and although I was on the fence about a website, I loved the idea of sharing my "secrets". The next morning (Labor Day 2017), I decided to write a book and quickly wrote the first two pages. I'm glad I ran into you that day, and I'm thankful for your idea, Preston!

*Dedicated to anyone who takes their health seriously;
to anyone who wants to know how a systematic, consistent,
non-drastic, common-sense approach to a healthy lifestyle
has worked for me, and how it can morph YOU into a fitter,
more youthful, more energetic, happier person.*

If you're ready to elevate yourself; this book is for you!

APPETIZER

"Who The *Hell* is Narc Narcisse?"
[PART I]

Chapter 1: The Beginning...

My mom, Jocelyne, was born and raised in Port-au-Prince—the capital of Haiti—in August, 1953. She lived there for the first twelve years of her life, until she moved across the Atlantic Ocean to Paris, France, in 1965. She spent her teenage years in the French Capital then in 1973 she migrated back across the pond to another big city—New York City—and eventually became a US citizen. At the age of twenty, my mother had just gone through her second cross-Atlantic move, enduring another major cultural and linguistic change in the process.

My dad, Jean, is also from Haiti—born and raised in Port-au-Prince, in September, 1948. He spent his entire childhood in the Caribbean nation. In the early 70s, in his mid-twenties, he moved to Paris. He stayed there for only a few years before he, too, migrated to the Big Apple. He got there in 1975 and ultimately became a US citizen, as well. His time in Paris was short but precious because that's when he met my mother.

Rumor has it, that's when Paris was nicknamed *The City of Love* and when the idea for the hit show "How I met your mother?" sprang to life!

Jocelyne and Jean reconnected in New York and became an item. Out of that union came me: born May 30, 1977, in Jersey City. My mom already had a daughter, Sandra—six years older than me—from a previous relationship, but I was my dad's first child. Most people think that *Narc Narcisse* is a fake name, or nowadays they may think it's my author name, but that's not the case. My dad gets the credit for *creating* my first name by using the first four letters of our last name, but my mom—after vetoing other suggested names—gets the credit for *accepting* it. For my parents, who had grown up in Haiti and France, the word "Narc" didn't have any special meaning or connotation with anything in particular; it just sounded cool and different.

Hence, Narc is not a nickname, not an alias, and not short for anything; it's my real and full first name given at birth.

After living in a small apartment in New York City until I was five years old, my dad, mom, sister, and I moved into a house in Jersey City, near Liberty State park. I was a tall, skinny, active kid who enjoyed playing sports, playing video games, and I absolutely loved watching *WWF* wrestling (today, known as *WWE*). I also liked school; I was an all-around good student, but math is where I really stood out. From day one, I was a natural, who excelled at it. #NerdAlert Math wasn't just my best subject, it was my *favorite* subject—it became part of my identity; I became known as "The Math Kid." My parents bragged about my math exploits whenever they could, especially during get-togethers with friends and family.

I went to school just a few blocks away from home, a Catholic school named Sacred Heart School. Many of our teachers were nuns, and they were quite strict. If you clowned around, you got your hand smacked with a wooden ruler— "Ouch!" Being a good student didn't prevent me from being a bit of an agitator at times; I may have gotten reprimanded once or twice... Ok, maybe a couple more times, but who's counting? At school, we had to wear uniforms daily: dark green pants; white or yellow buttoned up, long or short-sleeved shirts; a green tie; and a blazer. Wearing a uniform to school definitely made mornings much easier for my parents, as they didn't have to worry about what I was going to wear on a daily basis, but God forbid I spilled milk on my tie while eating breakfast—all hell broke loose!

On the surface, everything *seemed* relatively normal...

In addition to my older sister, on my mother's side, I also had two brothers—on my dad's side—who were slightly younger than me. I was born in May, 1977; my first brother, Nelk (another original name, courtesy of my dad), was born in October, 1977; and my second brother, Shawn, was born in December, 1977. Three sons born seven months apart??? [Insert thinking emoji] Yes, my dad had three sons from three different women the same year! What's even crazier is that everyone in the family knew about it, including my mom. Somehow, though, she stayed with him for nine more years...

I met my brother Shawn at a fairly young age; we got along really well. He spent time at my house in Jersey City, and my mom was very sweet to him. I also met Shawn's mom, and she was very sweet to me, as well. How and why were our mothers so accepting of the situation? I guess they weren't about to pass blame, anger, or any frustration on the kids. Now that I'm an adult, I can truly appreciate that behavior—it was highly commendable.

"What happened to Nelk, though, my *other* brother?"

We knew *of* him, but never met him during our childhood. His mother wanted nothing to do with my father or the Narcisse family as a whole. He grew up away from us and without knowing about our existence for two decades. We eventually met him in our early twenties; that day was surreal but amazing; it's not every day you got to meet your twenty-something-year-old brother from another mother—literally. Our personalities although distinct meshed really well; we all got along beautifully. It's been all smiles and laughs, ever since. I was even one of the two DJs at his wedding!

My dad lived with me, my mom, and my sister in Jersey City; consequently, he was a daily presence in my life. Shawn lived with his mom in Queens; to my dad's credit, despite the distance, he was very present in Shawn's life, too. Our dad knew he had done wrong, but he did do right by us, the kids.

In 1982, my dad had another child with a fourth woman. It was his first daughter; he named her Mozye (another original name). Again, everyone knew about it.

My mom wanted to keep the family together, so despite all the drama, she *still* stayed with him.

In May 1986, though, I'm not sure what happened, but my mom had enough and left my dad for good. She moved out of our house with Sandra and moved in with my grandmother in Manhattan. I was nine years old and in the third grade. School was still in session, so I continued to live at my dad's and attend Sacred Heart School as normal. My mom didn't drive (she still doesn't drive to this day), so on Friday evenings, my dad drove me to my Grandma's to spend the weekends there. He picked me up Sunday nights to take me back to our house in Jersey for the upcoming school week. This new routine went on for a little more than a month, until school was out for summer break mid-June. Ten days later my life was going to change drastically...

June 26, 1986.

That date is tattooed on my brain because the course of my life changed that day. It was a Thursday; my dad dropped me off at my grandma's for an extended weekend with my mom. As usual, when he dropped me off, he told me to have a good time; "I'll see you Sunday night, Son."

6

Shortly after he dropped me off, an uncle of mine arrived with a station wagon to pick up my mother, sister, grandmother, and myself. I still remember very vividly the large blue suitcases that were loaded in the back. Once we were all in the car, we sped off. My mom had picked out some nice clothes for me to wear and told me to change in the back seat—we were clearly in a rush. I asked my mom where we were going; what all the suitcases were for; and why I had to change clothes, in the back seat of a moving car, of all places. She told me that we were going on vacation. Looking out the windows, I noticed we were approaching John F. Kennedy airport. I had more questions:

"Where *is* this vacation?

What about dad?

What's going on?"

Although my mom tried to reassure me that everything was fine and that my dad knew about this, deep down I felt something wasn't right. She had perfectly choreographed that day. She arranged for my dad to drop me off at my grandma's by a certain time, she packed our luggage, she purchased the plane tickets, she got our passports ready, and she scheduled for my uncle drive us to the airport. To say that my mother is a strong, determined woman would be an understatement. But what if my dad had dropped me off late? What if, on our way to the airport, there was an accident on the freeway causing major traffic delays? What if the flight got canceled? So many things could have derailed my mother's master plan. But, in the end, everything went as planned: my mom, grandma, sister, and I got on a plane—it was headed to Paris, France. Once the plane took off, my mom had a huge sigh of relief. I didn't know it at the time, but this was no vacation...

My mom kidnapped me! I didn't see my dad or come back to the United States for the next three years...

[To Be Continued]

MAIN COURSE

"Why Do You Eat That Way?"

Chapter 2: My History with Food

As a kid, despite being super skinny, I was a big eater. I loved rice, pasta, steak, chicken, and spinach (thank you *Popeye the Sailor Man*). I also loved fast food, junk food, and sweets; hamburgers, French fries, pizza, hot dogs, potato chips, candy, cookies, donuts, cakes, and such were part of my food repertoire.

"How are my teeth not rotten?"

I was ecstatic when we took trips to McDonalds. My family always wondered how such a skinny kid could put away so much food, and so fast! Two Big Macs, large fries, six-piece chicken nuggets, and a large soda was my standard order; that was *my* version of a happy meal. I had a big appetite but was also quite picky and stubborn. I despised beans, which was a major problem because when you grew up in a Haitian household, beans were part of almost every meal:

- *Riz à pois rouge* (rice with red beans)
- *Riz à pois noir* (rice with black beans)
- *Riz à pois blanc* (rice with white beans)

"Are you serious?" I would sit there and take out EVERY single bean, one by one. And every time my siblings and cousins made fun of me, while my parents gave me the death stare.

"Can I just enjoy *my* rice the way *I* want to?"

Nope! My parents were annoyed with that behavior, to say the least. I remember one particular day, my mom told me that I could not leave the table unless I ate my beans. Five hours later, I was still camped at the table... What a stubborn punk! My mom, thankfully, gave up and just let me be. To this day, I still hate beans—yes, I know they are super healthy—and whenever I get together with my family, I'm still the only one who takes out every bean, one by one. Everyone just watches in amusement, while shaking their heads; "Same old Narc!"

Fast forward to college life. Despite being a Track & Field athlete, my nutrition was subpar. My dorm had healthy food options, but I always veered towards pizzas, burgers, fries, hotdogs, cheesesteaks, ice cream, donuts, sodas, etc. Back in the late 90s, McDonald's had a promotion on Tuesdays: two double cheeseburgers for $2.22. I was a BIG fan of that promotion and went almost every Tuesday. I generally ate SIX double cheeseburgers in one sitting. Yikes! I've always had a superfast metabolism, so despite all that eating, and all those bad calories, I was still skin and bones.

I joined the UCLA Track & Field team in 1998 as a 400m hurdler. I was a 6-foot-3-inch (1.90m) young man who weighed only 169 lbs (77 kilos). Ladies and gentlemen, *that* is what you call SKINNY. I competed relatively well, so I didn't think my nutrition was holding me back. I desperately wanted to put on muscle though; my coach wanted me to put on muscle, too. People made fun of me; they teased that I was too skinny and needed to eat more, not knowing how much I already ate.

I wanted to be buff since the age of fifteen; that's the age at which I joined my first gym. By my senior year at UCLA, I had "beefed up" to a meager 172 lbs (78 kilos). No matter what I did in the weight room, I simply wasn't making any gains. I graduated UCLA in the spring of 2001 and moved out of the dorms and into my first apartment that fall. For the first time in my life, I was responsible for feeding myself.

Cooking for yourself is a whole different ball game!

I didn't know how to make much besides white rice and plain pasta. I bought a George Forman grill and grilled steak, chicken, salmon, and ground beef. I also ate green beans, spinach, and broccoli; and for snacking I made ham and Swiss cheese sandwiches—that was it! I didn't know how to make anything else and was pretty content with my meals.

"You are what you eat," is NOT a myth!

My workouts hadn't changed, but my food was very different. I gained muscle, and it happened fast! I put on 8 lbs of muscle in my first month of cooking, and I was still super lean. I remember friends of mine asking me what kinds of *products* I was taking. I had been trying to put on muscles for almost ten years, and just like that, in a month, I packed on 8 lbs. I was in heaven! I realized it was my food that was making such a rapid impact, so I kept at it and continued to cook for myself. I began reading about nutrition and steadily improved my eating habits. I stopped drinking sodas and switched to water. I stopped eating ten cookies in one sitting, I stopped buying Doritos. I slowly reduced McDonald's (that wasn't easy). The gains kept coming! I went from 172 lbs to 180 lbs in a month, and then I slowly continued to gain muscle mass and remain extremely lean. I eventually reached 190 lbs, and then settled around 195 lbs. Twenty-three pounds of lean muscle in less than twelve months, all because I changed my eating habits. I was now being called BUFF; it felt awesome!

Funny story; I went to Paris to visit my mom during the summer of 2002, and when she saw me, she teared up. No, these weren't happy tears of a proud mom seeing her little boy all big and strong; they were sad tears because she thought I was taking steroids! She had last seen me at 172 lbs, and all of a sudden I was 195 lbs. I had to swear on my mother's life that I wasn't taking anything, that I was simply eating better.

"Wait. Did I really swear on my mother's life *to* my mother?"

My confidence increased tenfold. I now walked the streets with my chest out. If the sun was out, my *guns* were out! I got more attention from the ladies, too. I still remember the day a female friend complimented my butt. I didn't even know that was a good thing back then. My physical appearance improved but so did my athleticism. I actually became a better athlete years after my UCLA Track & Field Team days were over. Now, I am 40+ years old. Physically, I feel GREAT, and I look much younger than my age. My athleticism has not decreased; I may be even more athletic now than in my twenties. And for someone who's been an athlete since the age of fifteen, that's saying a lot!

Chapter 3: My Meals

Please remember that I'm a naturally very skinny person with a high metabolism, so my exact way of eating may not work for you, but I think there are still lots of points to take from my example.

Up until 2017, every morning, I used to have a bowl of cereal (Honey Bunch of Oats, from Costco) with yogurt (Original fruit flavored Yoplait). No milk with my cereal since I'm not a big fan, and yogurt with cereal tastes so good. I added mixed berries (from Costco) and açai powder in my yogurt. That combo made for quite a tasty and easy breakfast. I ate this EXACT same breakfast from 2002 until 2017, and I was very satisfied. Same cereal, same yogurt brand (different flavors), same berries, and same açai powder. When it comes to food, I am very unexciting. If I like it, I can eat the same thing every day and be happy.

I'm a weirdo. I know.

In January 2017, I changed my breakfast; that was quite a big deal after fifteen years. After hearing about the Ketogenic diet from a friend who had an amazing weight loss transformation, I was curious because I had simply never heard of it. I don't pay much attention to all these different diets, but after reading up on it, it caught my attention.

Let's back up a bit...

In September 2015, I got my body fat tested. I did a DEXA scan which is very accurate and thorough. I laid down on a table and my entire body got scanned (via X-rays) in ten minutes. It gave me a full breakdown of body composition (i.e. body fat and lean muscle mass) and informed me of the fat content in each limb, organ, and my trunk. It also measured my bone density and metabolic rate. After the scan, a nutritionist discussed the results with me. I did mine at **Bodyspec** for 50 dollars.

My body fat was 6.9%. I was pleased, but the nutritionist told me that was too low to just be walking around like that on a daily basis. She asked me about my food habits and suggested I add good fats to my diet—I listened and added avocados. I got rescanned in April 2016 and was at 7.1%; she said I was *still* too low and insisted I add MORE good fats. I was actually upset to have crossed into the 7% range, but I still figured that I should listen to her advice.

...Fast forward to 2017.

The ketogenic low carb diet is too extreme for me, but I nevertheless implemented an idea from it. The ketogenic diet has a love affair with eggs, and since the nutritionist *planted* the idea in my head (like the 2010 movie *Inception*) of adding more healthy fats to my diet, I made the decision (or was it *HER* decision?) to switch from a *carb*-loaded breakfast to a *fat*-loaded breakfast.

BREAKFAST

I now eat four organic scrambled eggs cooked in macadamia nut oil and seasoned with black pepper, garlic powder, and turmeric. I eat that with 2 slices of plain, untoasted white bread; I drink a small glass of 100% pure Pomegranate juice (from Whole Foods) and a tall glass of water.

LUNCH

I devour a huge plate of white Basmati or Jasmine rice (from Costco), sauced with *Heinz* Organic ketchup (zero GMOs and zero high fructose corn syrup). I've been eating my rice like that since I was a kid—I picked it up from my older sister. To my rice, I add broccoli, spinach, and asparagus (yes, all three every time), and half of an avocado.

For protein, it varies between steak, ground beef, and salmon.

- Mondays and Fridays: Steak
- Tuesdays, Thursdays, Saturdays, and Sundays: Salmon.
- Wednesdays: Ground Beef

Steak and ground beef are seasoned with black pepper and garlic powder. Salmon is seasoned with black pepper, garlic powder, and cayenne pepper. All three are grilled on my Ninja Foodi Indoor Grill—amazing piece of equipment! I finish off my lunch with a tall glass of water.

DINNER

I have the same white rice with ketchup, broccoli, spinach, asparagus, and the second half of the avocado.

For protein: chicken thighs, which are seasoned with black pepper, garlic powder, and chili powder. They're also grilled on my Ninja Foodi Indoor Grill. I finished off my dinner with a tall glass of water.

Let's talk about my protein selections

I purchase farmed salmon from the frozen section at Costco. I hear about the toxicity of farmed salmon, but I've yet to be convinced enough to stick to wild salmon—which is supposed to be healthier—and farmed salmon tastes so much better. I used to buy my other meats from Costco as well, which was convenient and financially efficient, but since early 2019, I decided to try organic, 100% grass-fed steak & ground beef and also organic, air-dried, skinless, boneless chicken thighs. I buy them all at Whole Foods; it's definitely more expensive, but the difference in taste alone is worth it for me—these meats are juicier and much more flavorful. Additionally, since the switch I feel even better. Consequently, organic, grass-fed meats have now become a staple in my nutrition.

SNACKS

I don't snack very often. My huge meals keep me full for hours at a time, but whenever I do get hungry between meals, I'll have either raw, unsalted almonds; walnuts; or if I need something more filling, I might indulge in chocolate croissants or even popcorn. Yup, there's nothing wrong with that once in a while. If I can get my hands on some decent crêpes, look out—they won't last long!

DRINKS

I love cold water; I drink it all day!

In the morning, I have a small glass of 100% pure pomegranate juice (not from concentrate and with no added preservatives). Not only does it taste amazing, but pomegranate is one of those super foods that everyone should be consuming regularly—I highly recommend it. Warning though: because it's naturally very sweet, I make sure I don't overdo it, which is why I stick to only a *small* glass in the morning.

Another drink that occasionally finds its way in my hands is Gatorade; maybe after a tough workout or something. In general, though, water is my go-to drink in most situations.

CHEAT MEALS

I get asked about this more than anything else. Once in a while, I eat pizza (a whole pie), crêpes, carrot cake, or even go on a late-night feeding trip to McDonald's or In N Out. If I'm coming back from partying and I'm hungry, you better believe that I'm going to eat something! At McDs, I typically have a Double Quarter Pounder with Cheese, large fries, 10-piece chicken nuggets with barbecue sauce, and a strawberry banana smoothie. At In N Out, I get two double-doubles and a cheeseburger. Whenever I eat like that, I don't feel one bit guilty because I know I eat well 85-90% of the time. I actually don't even like the word *cheat* meal because I don't feel like I'm cheating when I eat that way. I also don't feel the need to have a *built-in* "cheat" day in my routine. I can go on for weeks of eating my healthy meals and then have a weekend when I have two or three meals that don't fit my regular diet. No biggie! My daily meals don't feel restrictive to me—I believe that's key.

EATING OUT

Going to a fancy restaurant is not really a treat for me; it's often more of a chore. At any restaurant, as I scan the menu, my first thoughts are: "Is there any rice here? What about steak or chicken?"

When dining out, my favorite places usually include good rice. Cuisines from Thailand, Japan, China, and India are safe choices for me. PF Chang's is my go-to restaurant in my area. Their shrimp fried rice and sesame chicken or pepper steak (which both come with broccoli and bell peppers) are right up my alley. I order that same meal EVERY. SINGLE. TIME.

SPICES

Over the years, I've upped my spice game. I now use five spices daily: tumeric, black pepper, cayenne pepper, chili pepper, and garlic powder. Of those five, two are absolute rock stars in the spice game and should find their way on your foods, too.

- **Tumeric** is unanimously revered because of its main active ingredient: curcumin. Curcumin's powerful anti-inflammatory and very strong antioxidant properties are what make this spice a superstar, and thus an absolute must in anyone's spice arsenal. Tumeric is actually the newest member of my line-up; which begs the question: "What was I waiting for?" There is a caveat though; Tumeric contains only a very small amount of curcumin—around 3% by weight—and it is poorly absorbed into the bloodstream, unless it's consumed with black pepper, which enhances the absorption of curcumin by 2,000%.

  In summary, there won't be a drastic amount of curcumin consumed and absorbed when you spice your foods with Tumeric—which is why some people turn to curcumin supplements to get more—but I still like the idea of having this spice as part of my arsenal of spices; I just make sure I consume it with black pepper.

- **Black Pepper** has found itself on my foods ever since I was a kid. Back then I had no idea about its health properties; I just knew I liked its taste. Black pepper is another highly perceived member of the spice game. It is high in antioxidants, it has anti-inflammatory properties, and it boosts the absorption of nutrients like calcium, selenium, and turmeric, among others.

I know eating the way I do is unexciting, robotic, boring, and some may say abnormal. Many people treat food as a *guilty* pleasure. They enjoy variety and surprises; they enjoy experimenting and experiencing new foods, new flavors, and new recipes. Me, I've always enjoyed eating pretty much the same four to five meals—which drove my mother crazy growing up. I view food primarily as fuel that will affect my mood and energy.

I keep it healthy, keep it tasty, and keep it moving!

Chapter 4: My Do's

When eating, I try and follow certain principles while keeping things simple and efficient. Fueling my body with nutritious food keeps me energetic, healthy, and youthful. The six main nutrients essential to life are proteins, carbohydrates, fats, vitamins, minerals, and water. Each one has its purpose.

I DO make sure I get good quality protein in my meals.
Proteins are the primary building blocks of the body that make up muscle, bone, skin, hair, and many other tissues. Proteins from foods are broken down into their amino acids by the digestive system, which are then absorbed into the bloodstream and recombined to create over 10,000 different types of proteins that perform a vast array of functions in our bodies. Proteins are sources of energy; they provide 4 calories per gram, which can be used when there are not enough carbohydrates or fats. In general, though, **protein is NOT a wanted source of energy** because that leads to a breakdown of muscles and other important tissues.
I get high quality protein from my eggs, lean chicken thighs, lean steak, lean ground beef, and salmon.

MYTH BUSTER #1: "If you don't consume animal products, you will be protein deficient."
NOPE! I clearly have an affinity for animal-based proteins, but there are many high-quality non animal-based proteins in quinoa, lentils, beans, tofu, oatmeal, seeds, and many more. Therefore, being vegan and getting enough high-quality protein is not an issue, whatsoever.

I DO make sure I get carbohydrates (carbs) in my meals.
Carbs are the sugars, starches, and fibers found in foods. They provide 4 calories per gram; **carbs are the energy used first to**

fuel muscles and the brain. They can be grouped into two categories: simple and complex.

- Simple carbs (also called sugars) are glucose, fructose (fruit sugar) and galactose (milk sugar). Simple carbs are broken down quickly which lead to a spike in blood sugar and energy. *Natural* simple carbs such as those found in fruit need to be distinguished from their *non-natural* counterpart called *refined* carbs (or processed carbs). Refined carbs don't exist in nature in their processed form (e.g. table sugar, white rice, and white pasta). They come from natural whole foods, but they have been altered in some way by processing to *refine* them. Refined carbs get absorbed into the blood stream even quicker than natural simple carbs because they have been stripped down of important nutrients such as fiber and vitamins, which slow down absorption.

- Complex carbs consist of starches (large chains of glucose units) and dietary fiber. Starches are broken down much slower and thus release their glucose and energy at a much slower rate, which keep blood sugar levels lower and lead to sustained energy. Fiber provides little to no calories, but it is an absolute MUST for good health. It helps move food efficiently through the body during digestion, and it also slows down the absorption of sugars, which helps control blood sugar levels.

Rice is my main source of carbohydrates, but the fact that I eat *white* rice often raises questions: "Isn't white rice bad? Why not switch to brown rice?" many people ask me. White rice often gets a bad rap because of its highly refined carbs content and elevated glycemic index (GI). This index assigns a value (0 to 100) to foods that contain carbs, based on how slowly or how quickly those foods cause increases in blood glucose levels. Pure glucose is the reference point of the GI and was assigned the highest value of 100. In general, choosing foods with a low GI (under 55) is preferable, except when a quick burst of blood glucose and energy is needed such as during or right after a workout. The good news is that pairing high GI foods with other nutritious foods that have protein, healthy fats, and fiber (e.g. steak, salmon, broccoli, and avocado) will slow down the speed at which blood glucose rises and thus lower the overall glycemic *load* of your meal. This is why in many cultures, eating white rice is actually part of a healthy diet because of the way they combine their white rice with a nutritious diet, in addition to daily physical activity like walking.

MYTH BUSTER #2: "Carbs are bad, avoid them ALL to become healthier."
NOPE! Carbs are not created equal. **Not ALL carbs are bad.** Processed carbs should indeed be limited because of their lack of fiber, but even they can be useful when a quick rise in blood sugar (energy) is needed. Feeling a little light-headed after a workout? You might want to grab that cholate bar to get a quick rise in blood sugar. Just don't overdo it!

I DO make sure I get healthy fats in my meals.
Fats are required for proper functioning of our brain and our nerves; for maintaining healthy skin, hair and other tissues; and are part of countless other functions. Fats are also a major energy source, as they provide a whopping 9 calories per gram! When the body needs energy, fats are second in line (after carbs) to fuel the body. There are many types of fats: dietary fats (unsaturated, saturated, and trans fats), blood fats

(triglycerides), and cholesterol which is both dietary and blood fat.

- Triglycerides are blood fats made in the body from digesting and breaking down of fats from foods; they can also be made from other energy sources such as carbs. When you eat, your body converts any calories it doesn't immediately need into triglycerides, which then get stored in your fat cells for later use. When you are between meals and need energy, triglycerides get released to supply energy. They are important and needed, but if you regularly eat more calories than you burn, particularly from carbs and fats, your triglycerides count will be too high, and they will get stored in your hips, belly, and so forth.

- Cholesterol is a waxy, fat-like substance carried in the blood stream and is found in every cell of the body. It is used to make hormones, to make substances that help you digest foods, and also used to protect nerve cells—**Cholesterol is essential for life**. It comes from two sources: foods that contain animal fat, and it's also formed in the body (i.e. the liver). Plants contain no cholesterol. **It is important to note that even if you don't ingest a single gram of cholesterol, your body will still produce it every day, and may even produce it in excessive amounts.** When we talk about the different types of cholesterol, we are actually talking about the different types of *proteins* that carry cholesterol molecules through the bloodstream. LDL (low density lipoprotein) is usually referred to as "bad" cholesterol because it deposits its cholesterol on the walls of our arteries. This plaque buildup narrows arteries and raises the risk for heart attacks, strokes, and other artery diseases. HDL (high density lipoprotein) moves cholesterol safely throughout the body. It hangs on tightly to the cholesterol it carries and won't let it deposit on arterial walls. In some cases, it may even snatch up additional cholesterol already stuck to the wall, thereby reducing the size of a plaque buildup. For these reasons, HDL is considered to be the "good" cholesterol.

- Unsaturated fats are considered the *good* fats because they can improve blood cholesterol levels, stabilize heart rhythms, and play a number of other beneficial roles. They are predominantly found in fatty fish and in foods from plants (e.g. vegetables oils, avocados, nuts, and seeds). The most *popular* unsaturated fats are Omega-3 and Omega-6 fatty acids. These fatty acids are not simply stored or used for energy; they have important roles in processes like blood clotting and inflammation. **Omega-3s have an anti-inflammatory effect.** They are found in various foods (e.g. nuts, seeds, and grass-fed beef), but the forms found in fatty fish (e.g. salmon, herring, and sardines) are preferred. Omega-6s are found in certain vegetables oils, salad dressings, mayonnaise, snacks, etc. They are pro-inflammatory.

Inflammation is essential for our survival, it helps protect our bodies from infection and injury, but it can also cause severe damage and contribute to disease when the inflammatory response is inappropriate or excessive. Excess inflammation may be one of the leading drivers of the most serious diseases we are dealing with today (e.g. heart disease, diabetes, and Alzheimer's). The balance between Omega-3s and Omega-6s is believed to be a crucial element of optimal health. A diet that is high in

Omega-6s and low in Omega-3s increases inflammation (not good), while a diet that includes balanced amounts of each reduces inflammation (recommended).

- Saturated fats are considered the *bad* fat, but there are conflicting conclusions about its negative effects on health and, in particular, on heart health. Despite all the negative publicity, there still is no scientific evidence that *directly* links saturated fats to heart disease. In nature, they are mainly found in animal products (i.e. meats and dairy food), but can also be found in some plant sources such as coconut, palm oil, and cocoa butter. Saturated fats are also found in processed foods (i.e. fatty snacks, cakes, and deep fried foods).

- Trans fats are considered the *ugly* fat, because they raise your bad cholesterol (LDL) and lower your good cholesterol (HDL). Artificial Trans fats are created in an industrial process that adds hydrogen to liquid vegetable oil (i.e. *partially hydrogenated oils*) to make them more solid. Trans fats can be found in many fried foods and baked goods such as pastries, pizza dough, pie crust, and donuts.

I get high quality unsaturated fats from avocados and salmon. Steak, chicken and eggs have a high content of saturated fats. With so many conflicting studies about the true dangers of saturated fats, I am not convinced of their alleged danger. They have always been part of my meals and until further notice, they are here to stay. But if you are on the other side of the fence, limiting or eliminating these animal-based products may be the safe thing to do. No matter what, though, make sure you are getting unsaturated fats, especially the undisputed, healthy Omega-3s.

MYTH BUSTER #3: "Going on a low or no-fat diet is healthy; it will help me lose weight."

NOPE! ALL fats shouldn't be avoided at all cost. **Artificial Trans fats should be 100% eliminated, but healthy fats are essential to good health; especially Omega-3s!**

I DO make sure I eat my vegetables.

Your parents were on to something when they told you to eat your veggies, which provide you with vitamins, minerals, fiber, and antioxidants, while being naturally low in fat and calories. Vitamins and minerals are essential for life as they help regulate chemical reactions in the body. **Antioxidants are molecules that inhibit the oxidation of other molecules.** Oxidation is a chemical reaction that can produce free radicals (unstable molecules), leading to chain reactions that may damage cells.

Vitamins can't be made in the body (except for vitamin D, the *sunshine* vitamin), so we must obtain them through our diet. Minerals originate in the earth and cannot be made by living organisms. Plants absorb minerals from the soil, and animals get their minerals from the plants, or other animals they eat. Most of the minerals in the human diet come directly from plants, such as fruits and vegetables, or indirectly from animal sources. Minerals may also be present in natural water sources.

Fruits are also a great source of vitamins, minerals, fiber, and antioxidants, but they tend to be higher in sugar and calories.

MYTH BUSTER #4: "Orange juice is the best source of vitamin C."

NOPE! Red bell peppers actually have three times more vitamin C than oranges and more than the daily requirement of beta carotene (pro vitamin A).

SIDE NOTE: fruit juices and smoothies can sound like a great, healthy idea, but they tend to be low in fiber, which elevate blood sugar very rapidly. Also, because they are easy to binge drink, consuming too many calories and too much sugar at once is a lot easier than eating a whole fruit, which is much denser and thus fills you up much quicker. Proceed with caution!

I DO make sure I drink plenty of water throughout the day. Water, which has zero sugars and zero calories, is an essential nutrient because it is required in amounts that exceed the body's ability to produce it during digestion. The body can last a lot longer without food than without water. All biochemical reactions occur in water. It is required for digestion, absorption, transportation, dissolving nutrients, elimination of waste products, and regulation of body temperature through sweating. It also serves as a cushioning component between joints, in the spinal cord, and in the brain.

Water happens to be my favorite drink, so drinking it with my meals and throughout the day is very straightforward. **Staying hydrated is essential.** An easy way to track your level of hydration is by checking the color of your urine, which should be pale yellow instead of dark brown.

MYTH BUSTER #5: "Water has no taste."
NOPE! **When you stop binging on sugary drinks, your taste buds become alive and water actually starts to taste good—**I wouldn't lie to you! Make the switch, and before you know it, you'll be able to taste the difference between different brands of water and actually enjoy the *flavors*.

Chapter 5: My Don'ts

Sometimes, the best thing to do to accomplish a goal is to figure out what NOT to do. If you eliminate all bad habits, you'll be left with either no habits or, even better, with good habits. A diamond is quite ordinary at first, but its true beauty is only realized through the cutting, removal, and polishing process.

I DON'T drink sodas or soft drinks.
High sugar content and lack of nutritional value; need I say more? Foods that supply energy but contain very little or no nutrients are called empty calories. Sodas and soft drinks are classic examples of empty calories, which are the easiest thing to justify getting rid of for those seeking better health.
What about diet sodas? The diet version of sodas, at least brings down the calorie and sugar count, but still lack nutritional value. Opting for water instead is preferable, as it has zero calories, zero sugar, and is a nutrient on its own that helps every cell in your body function properly.

I DON'T drink coffee or energy drinks.
Not drinking coffee is not because of health concerns; it's simply not my thing. Black coffee actually has its place in a healthy diet. But when your energy drink or your morning hot flavored colorful latte from your favorite "coffee" shop has more sugar and calories in it than a can of soda, you have entered the non-healthy, empty-calorie zone. On a limited basis it should be okay but not part of a daily routine.

I DON'T add butter or oils to my foods.
This has nothing to do with health concerns since organic butter and certain vegetables oils in moderation are part of a healthy diet; it's just that I don't feel the need to do so. The meats and fish I eat have natural fats that add flavor and keep

them moist when grilled well (i.e. not over cooked). It's just a matter of taste, but for me, added oil or butter (even on my morning bread) is just too much.

Frying my eggs for breakfast is the only time I use oil at all, and I recently switched from olive oil to macadamia oil. Olive oil (Extra Virgin) is actually one of the healthiest oils out there—a staple of the Mediterranean diet—"So why the switch?" you may ask. Well, vegetable oils are not all created equal. There are two things to be aware of when selecting oils.

- If it's for cooking (e.g. frying eggs or steak, sautéing vegetables, etc.), **it's important to check the oil's smoking point.** The higher the temperature used for your cooking, the higher the smoking point of the oil should be to ensure it doesn't burn. Heating oil to the point where it begins to smoke, produces toxic fumes and harmful free radicals, which can cause damage to our cells. I used to fry my eggs with olive oil (smoking point 320 °F) and always noticed that the oil smoked and turned brown. But now that I've switched to macadamia nut oil (smoking point 390 °F), the oil does NOT smoke or turn brown anymore.

- Another important thing to watch for is the ratio of Omega-3 vs Omega-6 fats. Oils that have too much Omega-6s compared to Omega-3s or, even worst, that have zero Omega-3s should be avoided. More Omega-6s than Omega-3s is ok as long as the ratio is to not too skewed (i.e. more than a 4 to 1 ratio). Staying close to a 1 to 1 ratio is ideal. Avocado oil has the highest smoking point (520 °F) but has a 12 to 1 ratio of Omega-6s vs Omega-3s. So I've opted for macadamia nut oil, which has a high enough smoking point for my cooking needs and has a perfect 1 to 1 ratio of Omega-3s to Omega-6s.

31

I DON'T add salt to my food.

This is not because of any health concerns. I am by no means anti-salt. I just don't have a need for added salt. The verdict is still not clear if a high-salt diet is dangerous. For some people, though, a *too low* salt diet causes harm. Salt tolerance, as with most things, depends on the individual. The amount of daily salt one should consume to stay healthy varies greatly from individual to individual. The debate continues, so proceed with caution.

SIDE NOTE: when you stop many of the bad eating habits; your taste buds become alive, and you quickly realize that all that extra salt, extra sauce, extra sugar, or extra oil is no longer needed or wanted. I spice my foods with black and cayenne pepper, garlic, turmeric, and chili powder, which all add great flavors to my food and have health benefits—it's a win-win situation!

I DON'T drink milk or consume many dairy products.

As a kid, I drank low fat milk with my cereal because whole milk tasted horrible to me. As I grew older, I liked milk less and less and eventually switched to eating my cereal with yogurt. I haven't had a glass of milk in over fifteen years! I've always liked cheese, though, in particular Swiss cheese, but it's not part of my regular diet. Now that I've given up my morning cereal and yogurt in favor of eggs and bread, my diet is basically dairy free, except for the occasional cheese pizza, cheeseburger, or piece of cake. The more I read about dairy and its effects on humans, the more I am convinced that a non-dairy diet is the way to go. Could it be that humans as a species are lactose intolerant? [Insert thinking emoji]

I DON'T regularly eat desserts (e.g. cake, cookies, donuts, etc.), processed meats (e.g. bacon, hot dogs, and sausages), deep fried foods, pizza, and so forth.

These foods either have lots of processed sugars, lots of trans fats, or both! They are also part of the inflammatory foods list which is gaining more and more attention as being a big cause of many health issues including weight gain, skin problems, digestives issues, and a host of diseases from diabetes to obesity to cancer. Consuming these empty-calorie foods once in a while and in moderation won't do too much harm. But when it becomes part of a regular routine, your body will be in constant fight-mode to reduce the inflammation caused by these foods, which over time, leads to the issues listed above. I am by no means immune to the occasional trip to the fast food joint, to enjoying a slice or two of pizza (ok, maybe even the entire pie), or to having some pastries at a birthday party or wedding. I used to have a HUGE sweet tooth, which was basically an addiction. And, like most addictions, it takes time, effort and discipline to stop them. Now, many desserts are actually too sweet for me, and when I'm at home, dessert does not even cross my mind anymore—addiction defeated!

Not eating bacon has nothing to do with being health conscious. I stay away because of the strip of fat; I just can't put that in my mouth, as I've never been a fan of chunks of fat.

I DON'T weigh my food or count calories.

I've never even thought about doing that. People often ask me how many calories I eat per day, and I always give the same generic answer: "I don't know, but it's a lot... 5,000 maybe?" I cook balanced, nutritious meals and eat as much as I can until I'm full; then I wash it down with water. My food never makes me feel bloated or sleepy. It simply energizes me and gets me ready for the rest of my day. Good fuel equals good energy!

I DON'T eat out very often.

Cooking my own meals—and I don't mean simply heating up a pre-packaged, microwavable dinner—was a HUGE game changer. Cooking for myself was initially a daunting task. I had to spend time grocery shopping; I had to read labels in order to make good choices; and then I had to actually spend time cooking. But that gave me better control of the ingredients: how much salt, how much oil, what *type* of oil, how much sauce, how much added sugars, etc.

Seeing rapid changes in my body composition fueled my motivation to keep it up. No need to be a chef to make simple, healthy, and tasty meals. It just takes a little effort, discipline, proper planning, and good quality Tupperware. I make my rice and vegetables in bulk (i.e. about four days' worth at a time). At all times, in my refrigerator there is one Tupperware with rice, one with broccoli, one with asparagus, and one with spinach; I also have avocados on deck. When it's time to eat, I fill my plate with rice and vegetables then microwave for four-and-a-half minutes while I grill my meat or fish. The whole process is quite speedy; it usually takes me about fifteen minutes from the minute I decide to cook to actually being seated in front of my plate, ready for action. I'm all about being healthy, but efficiency and convenience are very important to me, as well.

DESSERT

"Can I Have That Last Piece?"

Chapter 6: You Shouldn't Do That, You Should Do This

YOU SHOULDN'T be pressured to change your physical appearance because of peer pressure, because of some need to fit in, because of the latest trend, because some weirdo named Narc is telling you to, etc. If you're satisfied with your current health, current physique, current level of energy, etc. then well done, keep doing what you're doing!

YOU SHOULD make changes to your eating habits if YOU feel the desire to improve your health, if YOU feel the desire to change your appearance, if YOU want to raise your energy levels, and so forth.

Many people made fun of me when I was super skinny, somehow I didn't let it get to me. Me wanting to get buff was never a peer pressure thing, a revenge thing, or a need to fit in. I just wanted muscles because I had a vision of myself. I realize that today with social media, Instagram in particular, it's very difficult to avoid the comparisons, and to avoid thinking you need to do this or that to fit in. **Don't do it for the Gram; do it for YOU!** Whatever you choose, do it because you truly want to, not because it's trendy. If a particular trend didn't exist or suddenly stopped being trendy, would you still want to do it? If the answer is yes, you my friend are doing it for the right reason. Keep on keeping on!

YOU SHOULDN'T be obsessed with losing weight if your true goal is to lose fat. Losing weight is actually quite simple. It's just a matter of eating fewer calories than you burn per day. Yes, it's that easy! If you burn 2000 calories per day and eat 1800 calories per day, you will lose weight no matter where those calories come from. But where will the weight loss come from? Will it be a decrease in body fat, shrinkage of muscle tissue, loss of water, or the dreaded deterioration of bone mass? You DO NOT want to be promoting a reduction in bone mass or bone density. Your bones need proper fuel to stay strong; this becomes even more important as you age. Bone health is crucial! A great diet promotes overall health and helps your body fight illnesses.

YOU SHOULD worry about keeping your body fat low. It is much wiser to worry about your body fat percentage. Be aware that the scale can sometimes be your worst enemy. You can go from 30% body fat to 22% body fat but actually weigh more, because if you burned fat and added muscle, your overall weight might actually go up since muscle weighs more than fat. But your body shape and size will change; you will be slimmer and more toned despite weighing more. So don't let the scale be the ONLY judge of your progress. Body fat percentage is a much better indicator of progress.

My advice to those seeking weight loss, but really want to lose fat, should consider checking their body fat percentage. DEXA scans are amazing, thorough, and quick. Leave the dramatic scale weigh-ins to the Mayweathers and McGregors of the world, and worry primarily about lowering your body fat percentage. And don't be surprised if you actually appreciate your weight gains because it came via a reduction in body fat AND a more toned body. You won't talk about weight *loss* goals anymore; it will simply be about GAINS or GAINZ with a Z if you're about that life!

YOU SHOULDN'T make changes that are so drastic that keeping up with them will be extremely difficult. Crash diets to get that summer body in a few weeks can work, but what happens after the diet is over? Will you *yoyo* back to your previous self? Will you feel absolutely miserable during the diet?

YOU SHOULD make gradual changes that will be much easier to keep up with. One step at a time is a cliché for a reason; it works! Instead of crash dieting, it's better to make changes that become part of your normal routine. Your taste buds will change, your energy will change, you will no longer have to get ready for summer; you will be ready year-round! There are many diets out there, low-fat, low-carb, no-fat, no-carb, raw foods, juicing, vegan, etc. Some of those diets work extremely well, but if you can't sustain it for the long haul, I think you're missing the true point.

This is obviously my opinion, but I believe making your daily eating habits something you can sustain 80-90% of the time is the way to go. You'll realize that you start making good choices naturally without it feeling restrictive. When that happens, you my friend will be a full-fledged member of the club! The club where a good, healthy meal sounds more appealing than a value meal at the local fast food joint. Get ready to answer lots of questions about your appearance, your high energy, and youthful appearance. You might even write a book about it!

Last but not least...
YOU SHOULDN'T blindly believe everything in this book, on Netflix, on the internet, and so on. What if I'm a fool who has no clue what I'm talking about? What if I'm biased and can only see things one way? What if I'm a fraud, who is taking money from certain companies to promote their brand?
YOU SHOULD question everything! There is so much misinformation out there; doing your due diligence should be standard practice. Do your own research, educate yourself, and meet with professionals (i.e. doctors, nutritionists, and dieticians). And as always, proceed with caution!

Chapter 7: My Final words

My goal is to live healthy, stay youthful, and be happy. Genetics and eating habits make for a powerful combination that will affect all three of those things.

Genetics are given, but diet is chosen.

My diet is far from perfect, and frankly I am not seeking THE perfect diet. My goal is to be balanced. I want good healthy foods that I *actually* enjoy eating, that are straightforward to cook, that are easy to shop for, and that are within my budget. As far as organic options are concerned, if they are easy to find, and at a price that I am comfortable with, then sure I grab them. When I wrote the first version of this book in 2017, I didn't stress about it too much. Now, almost two years later, I've upgraded to organic and 100% grass-fed meats, but I still eat many foods that don't fall into those two categories. As I continue to educate myself, someday, I may upgrade to eating *only* organic foods; someday, I may even decide to become a vegetarian or even a vegan. The door is always open... Years ago I took control of my diet and never looked back.

Take control of your diet; the power is in YOUR hands!

You can start by making some small changes to your daily eating habits. Remember, there is no perfect diet. There are many styles of nutrition that suit different people depending on their genetics, cultural habits, preferences, and so forth. Ideally, if, and when, you do decide to make changes, you do it in a way that it becomes a lifestyle rather than some intense crash diet that is unsustainable for the long haul. Realize that even starting *small* is already half the battle because you STARTED.

Ditch that soda or sugary juice, and opt for water instead. Say no to that morning sugar-filled latte and swap it for black coffee (in moderation of course). Eat more healthy fats such as Omega-3s by eating more fish. Double check the vegetable oils you use (Omega-3s vs Omega-6s ratio and smoking point). Add vegetables to your meals. I repeat ADD VEGETABLES TO YOUR MEALS. Fruit juice and smoothies are not the same as eating whole fruit. Eliminate trans fats and limit refined sugars by skipping daily desserts and unhealthy snacks. Avoid processed foods; they tend to be high in processed sugars, low in nutrients, low in fiber, full of artificial ingredients, trans fats, etc. Dine out less and stop ordering takeout everyday; you will expose yourself to less processed foods.

Start cooking your own meals, it's a game changer!

Need I say more? You have so many ways to make strides. See a professional: a health coach, a nutritionist, or a dietician. Treat your health and your body as if it was a highly sophisticated machine... Oh, wait. It actually is!

What about physical activity you may wonder: "Should I be doing something?" Umm, yes, you should! Let me explain...
[To be continued #Vol. 2]

About The Author

Narc Narcisse was born in Jersey City, NJ; raised in Paris, France; and currently resides in Los Angeles, Ca. He has a Bachelor of Science Degree in Physics from UCLA (class of 2001). He's been an athlete for 25+ years, a sports coach for 17+ years, and a teacher (primarily Physics) for 15+ years. He was a member of the UCLA Track & Field team and competed internationally in the long jump for Haiti at the Pan American Games in 2007. He has taught at Brentwood School (Physics & French) and Milken Community Schools (Physics & Chemistry). He currently coaches Cross Country and Track & Field at Brentwood School in Los Angeles.

Narc—a self-declared nerd—is not a nutritionist, a dietitian, or a doctor, but he knows a thing or two about being fit and healthy. He's a health enthusiast who uses his science skills to do research, his teaching abilities to educate, and his coaching tactics to motivate. Since September 2017 (Labor Day)—fueled by his desire to help people become the best version of themselves—he has ventured into the world of writing and publishing. Totally unrelated, he's also a DJ... You can't make this stuff up, can you?

Inspire, Inform, Empower

Thank you for reading.

This book is now finished.

Or is it...?

Inspire, Inform, Empower

You're STILL here?

Are you *really* expecting a post-credits scene?

This is NOT a Super Hero movie.

It's over, bye.

Inspire, Inform, Empower

Post-Credits Menu: Food For Thought

I owned the same car from 2001 to 2018. People were always surprised to hear that, and even more surprised when they saw it because it didn't look too bad. I was often asked how I kept it for so long. It was a simple answer: "I took care of it!"

If I were to tell you that the next car you get, you will have to keep for 17 years, I have a feeling you would take great care of it, too. You'd make sure you keep up with the maintenance, make sure you change the oil when needed, make sure you stay on top of the engine fluids, make sure you rotate the tires, and so on. And if a warning light came on, you'd bring it in to your mechanic to get it checked, right?

Let's get even crazier and say you have to keep your current cell phone for ten years!

Sounds impossible, right? Well, what if you absolutely HAD to because you simply couldn't get another phone for a decade. You would most likely buy a nice protective case for it, you would make sure you charge the battery with a proper charger to maintain the battery life, you wouldn't download random apps, you wouldn't go to random websites in fear of viruses, etc.

Usually, the longer you have to keep something and the more difficult it is to replace, the better you will take care of it...

How LONG do you intend to keep YOUR body?

[Insert thinking emoji]

Now, it's over...

BYE FELICIA!

www.ingramcontent.com/pod-product-compliance
Lightning Source LLC
Chambersburg PA
CBHW020407290526
45785CB00005B/2460